Table of Contents

The information in this Book is not intended to be a replacement for professional medical advice, diagnosis or treatment. Always seek the advice of your GP or other certified health representative with any questions about your medical condition. Do not disregard professional medical advice or delay seeking advice or treatment because of something you have read in "Mother's Secrets For A Healthy Winter". The contained in this Book is provided 'as is' without warranty of any kind. The entire risk as to the results and the performance of the information is assumed by the user, and in no event shall MyTeaSpoonOfHealth.com be liable for any consequential, incidental or direct damages suffered in the course of using the information in this Book.

"All That Man Needs For Health and Healing Has Been Provided

By

God in Nature,

The Challenge Of Science Is To Find It."

Philippus Aureolus Theophrastus Bombastus von Hohenheim – Aureolus Paracelsus (1493-1541)

MOTHER'S SECRETS FOR A HEALTHY WINTER

Introduction

Hello, my name is Rosalie and I am a mother of one gorgeous little girl.

My first thought every morning when I wake up is:

"Thank You! My Daughter Is Healthy"

To be a parent is a miracle.

To feel this precious soul and touch the tiny fingers……... and hold the little body of your child is heavenly satisfying.

I always feel grateful and blessed when I look at my little daughter.

She is the most beautiful, polite, kind, caring, smart, talented, and unique child in the world. She is my Sun, Oxygen, Water, and Air.

She is my Happiness!

I am sure you feel the same when you look at your little descendant or even think about her or him. The warmth and joy that fill up your heart are endless and you want them to stay forever there.

Our children are the most precious gifts and we want them to be always healthy, happy, and satisfied. We always look for ways to provide for their safety, meet their material needs, create great emotions and various activities, and give them all the love in the world.

We want them to have everything they deserve and enjoy growing up with plenty of support and love.

We want them to be full of energy and keep the house muddled (toys, books, pencils, drawings, even candies all over the house).

Although at times we raise our voices at them to clean up the chaos, we are happy and grateful that they have the strength to do it soooooo messy.

Yes, every parent has a different opinion about how, when, and why to educate his/her child, however, we all wish them to be healthy and happy.

We all want our children to be strong and well. Sometimes though we feel scared and helpless when our little treasure is getting cold or feeling sick.

My nightmare is ………. Colds, Flu, Viruses, High Fever….

Was my nightmare…………

But Not Anymore!

I have been trying various recipes and discovered a few unique mixtures that are helping me stop the nightmare from the first sneeze.

I wish to share my experience with you and help you see different ways to fight your nightmares.

In this book, I am going to tell you a few stories about myself and my encounters with herbs.

I will share with you some recipes that I discovered during the process of helping my family stay healthy, and energized and enjoy great times.

I am honestly grateful to all the natural goods that helped me keep my child well and strong, while friends, neighbors, and colleagues complained of flu, colds, and lack of energy.

This book is for people like you and me, who are not specialists and enjoy using herbs and plants in their daily meals only to enhance the taste and the benefits of the dish.

I have been collecting this information and experienced all the recipes throughout the years and I would love to share my knowledge with you.

Chapter I: A Little Bit About the Herbs

Herbs can be used in the forms of teas, syrups, oils, salves, tinctures, herbal pills, baths, poultices, and compresses. All the herbs and natural remedies are a gift from our land. I am sure that you are grateful same as me to nature for providing us with this amazing inheritance.

"Until man duplicates a blade of grass, nature can laugh at his so-called scientific knowledge. Remedies from chemicals will never stand in favor compared with the products of nature, the living cell of the plant, the final result of the rays of the sun, the mother of all life." – T.A. Edison

My story started many years ago when I was still in third grade. I always loved the fresh and innocent aroma of flowers and herbs (I guess my parents knew very well when they named me Rosalie).

We used to live in the city, in an apartment in just newly developed residential area. Behind our building was an open field, grass, flowers, playgrounds, and trees. I loved to play there with my friends.

During one of our school summer vacations, my friend and I heard that a local company purchases herbs. We did not know exactly what they used to do with these herbs, either we know what they looked like.

Anyway, we got the list of herb names and started the journey…... I found one book at home (my parents' library) about herbs and searched the names from the list.

That time I discovered the Common Mallow which is used traditionally as an herbal remedy for asthma, bronchitis, coughing, and throat infections….

I guess my first "summer salary" came from herbs. The most important is that I discovered the magic planet of herbs and plants and spices………

We all know that once scientific research started and chemistry was discovered, the battle between nature and chemicals began.

AND

We all know that the dispute between chemistry and nature is almost won in favor of NATURE.

You know that Herbalism (herbal treatment) is as old as mankind.

What is different from before and now is that humans changed their methods of using herbs throughout their evolution. The methods are different and improved because of the human experience and combination of folk medicine in every country.

There are thousands of biochemical reactions in our bodies. And when they are all normal, the metabolism in our body performs properly. When that happens, it is believed that the body is healthy.

I MUST emphasize that herbalism is recommended as a complementary therapy that comes in support of official medicine and that is matched correctly and competently with the rest of the treatment.

In the book I am giving you information on how far the possibilities are of herbal treatments for diseases or conditions which cannot be relied upon or to be combined with other treatments.

So, let us begin……………….

Chapter II: My Favourite Herbs I Use To Beat Colds and Flu

"I believe that there are many herbs and many trees that are worth much in Europe for dyes and for medicines; but I do not know, and this causes me great sorrow. Arriving at this cape, I found the smell of the trees and flowers so delicious that it seemed the pleasantest thing in the world." – Christopher Columbus

Basil – Osimum Basilicum

One of my favorite herbs. I love it, I love it, I really love it……..

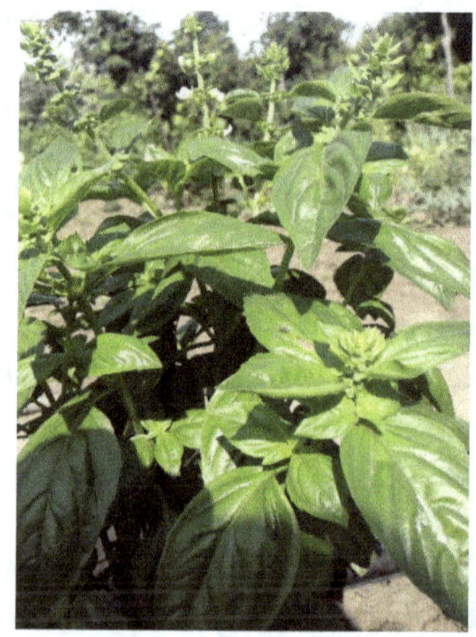

Basil is connected to many myths and legends……… In India, Basil is "doomed" to the God Vishnu, because it protects the terrible mythical serpent that "kills eyes". In Egypt, it was used to embalm the dead. During the Roman Empire served sprig of Basil was a sign of expressing love. In Mexico, it was thought that if you wear a sprig of Basil in your pocket, it will bring you money and your loved one will be forever faithful.

Did you know that...

Basil is an annual herb with a characteristic pleasant aroma. The stem is 20-60 cm high, four-ribbed branching from the base. The leaves are opposite, ovate, rarely toothed, with long petioles.

The flowers are white or pinkish-purple, arranged in groups of 6 in the bosoms of leaves, with 5-leaf whorl and 4 stamens. The fruit is dry and crumbles 4 brownish black monocotyledon smooth or grained nuts.

It blooms in July and August. For remedy are used the stems of Basil (Herba Basilici).

Overhead parts or stems of the plant are collected during flowering (July). You can cut some portion of the stem with some leaves, so they can grow new stems. The dried herb should have a light green color and white flowers, a distinctive smell, a slightly peppery flavor, and a maximum moisture content of 12%.

The Basil's home is the tropics of Asia and Africa. But has been cultivated in Europe for centuries. It was really valuable in ancient Greece, Egypt, and India.

I am sure you heard that in India is called Holy Basil. Some studies by Indian professionals show that the Holy Basil plant has antioxidant properties and helps the body fight the aging process. So, let us learn more about this blessed herb.

What is its chemical composition?

Basil oil has various chemical compounds that include a-pinene, camphene, b-pinene, myrcene, limonene, cis-ocimene, camphor, linalool, methyl chavicol, y-terpineol, geraniol, methyl cinnamate, and eugenol.

Basil remedies contain 0,02 to 0,50% essential oil (linalool, methyl chavicol, cineole, eugenol, geraniol, ocimene, sesquiterpen), 5% tannins, saponins, and little flavonoids.

Health Benefits

Basil has antiseptic, antispasmodic, analgesic, anti-inflammatory, and slightly exciting action. It is used in infectious inflammation of the urogenital and respiratory tract, fatigue, and depression.

Externally, it is used to impose skin rashes and swelling.

According to folk medicine, juice from fresh leaves of Basil is used in acute suppurative otitis media (ASOM), as well as difficult healing wounds.

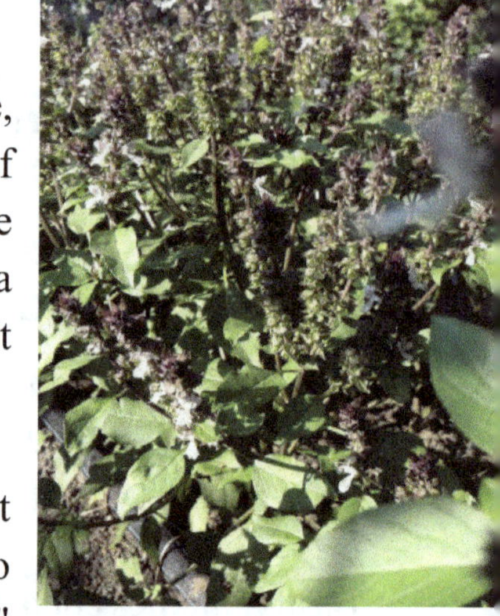

Excellent tool against mosquitoes. The best way to send these little "vampires" away is to have little bushes of Basil around your house or potted Basil attached to the window or the door.

You can prepare

2 tablespoons of the herb added to 300 ml boiling water, boil for 1 minute. Soak for 10 minutes, strain it, and drink 3 times daily before meals.

This tea is one of my remedies when we catch a cold with a cough.

Other uses of the herb

Basil is widely used in the cuisine of Southern nations, where due to the warm climate the food gets quickly spoiled. They use the preservative and antiseptic properties of the essential oils in Basil.

In cooking is an essential ingredient in many dishes from Italian cuisine to spice roasted beef and poultry; for preparation of broths and marinates; added into balsamic vinegar (in combination with tarragon and dill); fresh Basil in salads and dishes from fish and eggs………

Only imagine the steaming pizza Margarita…………… Crispy crust, tomato slices, melted mozzarella, and FRESH BASIL on top to finish the magic……………. Yummy, right?!

And of course, the famous pesto. This creamy mix made of fresh Basil, nuts, parmesan, and olive oil is delicious. You can make it, store it in a small glass jar, and keep it in the fridge for up to 2 weeks. Then use it for salads, pasta, pizza, roasted chicken…... Any dish you wish to prepare will be happy to receive a spoonful of this delight 😊.

And of course, don't forget to send away the unwanted nuisances, while enjoying your evenings in the garden.

Health Risk

Attention! Adopted in large quantities herb is toxic!

Although Basil oil usually stimulates, in excess it can have a stupefying effect and should not be used during pregnancy or on children under 16 years.

Since it can irritate sensitive skin, it must be used with care on people with such skin. It also has emmenagogue properties (emmenagogues are substances that can provoke menstruation), so it must be avoided during pregnancy.

Now, take a break, get up, and make some Basil pesto…….

The Best Pesto Ever:

Ingredients:
1 Cup fresh Basil leaves
2 tablespoons pine nuts, toasted
1 clove garlic
2 tablespoons Parmesan cheese
¼ cup extra-virgin olive oil
Himalayan or kosher salt and black pepper

Place the garlic, pine nuts, Basil, ½ teaspoon salt, and ¼ black pepper in the bowl of a food processor and pulse to combine. While the machine is running, drizzle in the olive oil, stopping occasionally to scrape down the sides. Transfer to a bowl and stir in the Parmesan.

Enjoy the pesto with some linguine or just spread it on a toast.

With The Best Pesto Ever on Toast, my daughter had lunch today. She added some fresh tomato and cucumber salad to the delight and experienced the bliss… 🙂.

Chamomile – Matricaria Chamomilla

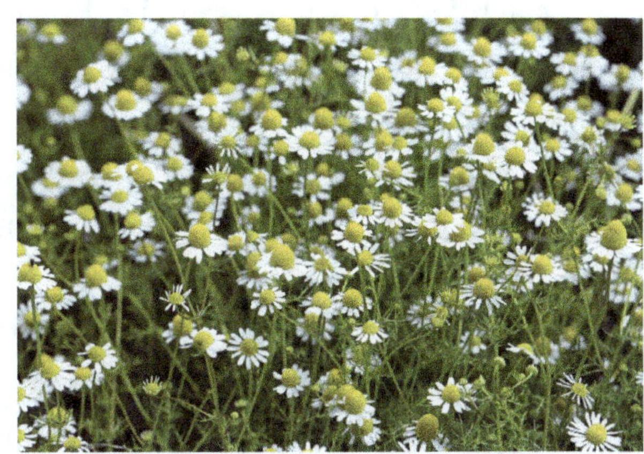

This is my favorite daily remedy. With its delicate and gentle flavor, I use it for almost everything – soothing, relaxing, calming, and of course anti-inflammatory…. Even the ancient Egyptians gave great attention to this marvelous herb and prescribed Chamomile tea as a cold remedy.

Did you know that…

Chamomile is an annual herb with branched stems 50 cm high. The leaves are double to triple pinnate, filamentary, and chopped.

The flower baskets are located on the top of many stem ramifications on long stalks and consist of white ring tabs female flowers and internal angular, yellow hermaphrodite flowers.

The torus is convex, and inside – hollow (typical of Chamomile). The fruit is an oblong brown seed.

The plant occurs through meadows, glades, and along roads throughout the country.

The herb is the flower of Chamomile – Flores Chamomillae.

The flower baskets with detachable small parts of stems are collected during flowering (May – July) and arranged in shallow baskets. They are dried up in the shade or the oven. The dried baskets have white gum leaves, and the cups and handles are green. The herb has a pleasant smell and slightly bitter taste.

What is its chemical composition?

The Chamomile flower contains essential oil, which has a green to blue color depending on the amount of azulenes. The oil has a large quantity of paraffin, caprylic, nonyl, and isovaleric acid.

The herb contains coumarins, mucus components, salicylic acid, nicotinic acid, linoleic acid, carotene, vitamin C, mucus, and bitter substances.

Health Benefits

The rich composition of the herb and the essential oil determines the multiple operations and uses of the herb. The essential oil of Chamomile has anti-inflammatory and softening effects in diseases of the digestive tract – colic in the stomach and intestines, gastritis, colitis, and inflammation of the respiratory tract – tonsillitis, pharyngitis, laryngitis (inhalation with oil steam).

External is applied as a wash in inflammation of the eyes. It has a beneficial effect on inflammatory processes and kidney stones and bladder.

The essential oil increases the number of cardiac contractility and expands the vessels of the brain.

You can prepare

The infusion of flower baskets of Chamomile improves and accelerates tissue regeneration therefore is used in difficult healing wounds in the form of compresses.

You can use the hot infusion for bronchial asthma, allergic gastritis, ulcers, and colitis, epilepsy, and headache. Compresses you can use for wet eczema, burns, swellings, boils, sweating of the feet, and uterine bleeding.

I prepare the cold extract by using 10 teaspoons herb and cover them with 2 glasses of cold water.

I leave it for 8 hours to extract, and then I strain it.

To make the infusion, cover 1 tablespoon herb with 200 ml boiling water. Soak it for 1 hour and the strained infusion you should take at once. Usually is taken 3 times a day, however, the infusions are prepared fresh each time.

Other uses of the herb

You can use Chamomile to provide skin relief if you need to. Rub the crushed flowers on the skin as a cosmetic. The Egyptians could not find a more beneficial ingredient in embalming oil to preserve deceased pharaohs.

You may rinse your mouth with Chamomile too to defy mouth sores.

Chamomile tea is the perfect solution to hold on to your little joys and have relaxed feet.

Health Risk

None that I know of………

The Most Soothing Tea In The World:

OK, enough chatting……..... Go make a cup of this wonderful tea and enjoy its seamless flow of relaxation and mindfulness.

Common Mallow – Malva Sylvestris L, Malva Vulgaris

This is the first herb I met when I was around ten and it sparked my love for herbs. Mallow is used traditionally as an herbal remedy for asthma, bronchitis, coughing and throat infection and I count on it when needed.

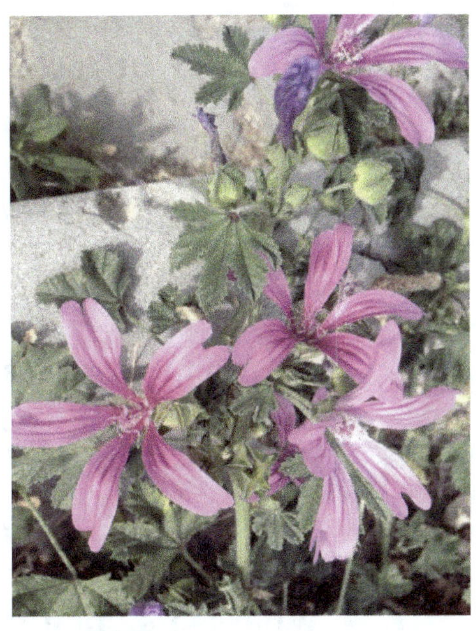

Did you know that...

The sort is native to the eastern Mediterranean and North Africa, but is now naturalized in many parts of the world.

Mallow is a biennial or perennial plant of the Malvaceae plant family. It is covered with small hairs and usually has creeping stems. It can grow up to one meter in height.

The leaves are dark green, and the flowers are pink with purple darker veins (the flower of Mauritanian mallow are deep purple). The flowers are 2 to 5 cm wide and the petals are three to four times longer than the cup.

The fruit is ring-shaped and splits into many smaller seed.
Broad-leaved Mallow can be found in gardens to villas and houses, as well as the green city zones.

What is its chemical composition?

It's especially rich in mucus substances and the flowers of these substances are therefore used extensively in herbal medicine. Although the fresh herb incorporates a lot of mucilage, it is destroyed when is dry. So, if you are looking for healing characteristics of mucilage, you should eat it fresh.

The leaves and flower buds contain mucus, tannins, flavonoids, essential oil, Vitamin C, Pro-Vitamin A and other substances. The anthocyanin glycoside malvin, a naturally occurring chemical, is only found in the flowers.

Health Benefits

As I mentioned already, Mallow is used as an herbal remedy for asthma, bronchitis, coughing, throat infections and emphysema.

It is also used to treat wounds or inflammation of the mucus membrane in the mouth, throat, stomach and intestines. The herb contains lots of mucous substances that cover the inflamed tissue with a protective layer.

Other uses of the herb in traditional herbal medicine include the treatment of gallstones, kidney stones, kidney inflammation, headache, constipation, gastritis, inflammatory diseases of the liver, toothache and insomnia.

     MOTHER'S SECRETS FOR A HEALTHY WINTER

You can use Mallow externally to treat wounds, boils, insect bites, eczemas, skin rashes, swellings, pimples... Be thankful to its bactericidal, astringent and anti- inflammatory properties.

You can prepare

As cough remedy you can prepare tea – take 2 tea spoons of leaves or flowers and cover with 400 ml lukewarm water. Leave it for 3-5 minutes, strain and drink.

If you wish to make infusion (stronger than the tea), allow the flowers or the leaves to soak for few hours in lukewarm (better cold) water, then strain and drink.

Please do not boil the herb, because all the medical greatness will go away.

It is believed that the herb cures even extremely stubborn and incurable lung emphysema, which sometimes causes strong shortness of breath.

In these cases, drink at least three cups a day

OR

Make a compress: Well strained and warmed leaves and flowers are placed for the night on your chest in the area of the bronchi and lungs.

The herb is used for baths and gargles too. Chilled decoction of Mallow you can place on the eye against drying.

Other uses of the herb

These days, the dried flowers and extracts are used in many commercial tea blends and cough syrups. The root can be used as a toothbrush 😊

Mallow tea is recommended as well to nursing mothers to help them produce more milk. Malva Sylvestris has delicious seeds, which taste similar to young hazel nuts and they can be easily included in green salads along with the leaves and flowers.

The use of common Mallow in the kitchen is mostly forgotten, but absolutely deserves to return back.

Health Risk

There are no known side effects from the herb when it is used in prescribed doses.

The Forgotten Salad Garnish:

I hope that the Mallow is in season now in your area, so GET OUT and find it. Try the "cheese wheels" right there and take few leaves, flowers and seeds of course.

Wash them well, pat dry with paper towel and add them to your choice of salad.

Enjoy this nutritious, tasty and refreshing meal.

Elderberry – Sambucus Nigra

I thought that only the goats eat these violet-black small fruits taking them directly from the bush……

I was wrong!

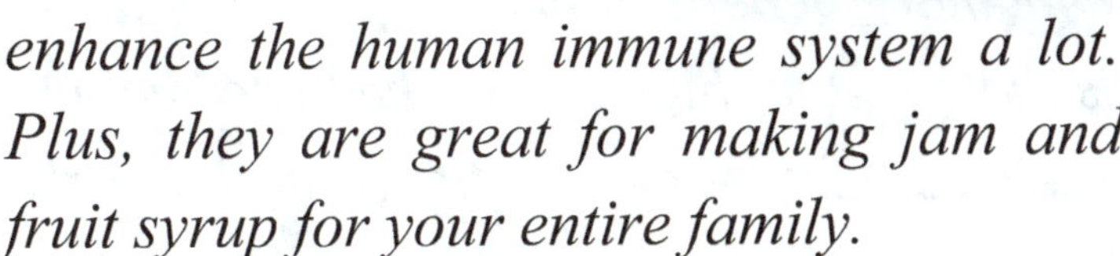

These fruits are full of Vitamins and they enhance the human immune system a lot. Plus, they are great for making jam and fruit syrup for your entire family.

Last summer I made marmalade only from the fruits, without any sugar or sweetener. The best part was that my daughter helped me collect, clean, and extract the juice from the fruits 😊*.*

If you try, make sure you use gloves…… We did NOT and for the next week, we had dark violet-black fingers and "natural" nail polish with the same color…… 😊😊😊.

However, we had a marvelous time preparing the marmalade and during the winter, when we opened the first jar, we could not stop enjoying the memories of the summer.

One more benefit of making it by ourselves is that my daughter enjoys the taste because she was part of the creation. And honestly, she prefers our sugar-free jam to the one bought from the store……

Did you know that...

The plant is a shrub or tree with spreading branches and a white foam core.

The leaves are cloven-pinnate with 2-3 pairs of leaflets, long up to 20 cm. The individual leaflets are ovate and oblong, tapered, densely serrated.

The flowers are very small, yellowish-white, collected outerwear complex inflorescences. The stamens are five, with large yellow anthers.

The plant is ubiquitous in moist places, around the undergrowth, in forests, and in settlements.

The flowers and the fruits are collected and used as herb–Flores at Fructus Sambuci.

Rarely are used the roots and the inner bark of the stem. The flowers are picked in dry and sunny weather before their full blossoming (May – June). They are dried immediately in the shade or a dryer. The dried flowers are yellow-white, with a pleasant aroma. Once dried, the herb is sifted through a dense sieve, through which pass only blooms, but the small flower stalks remain non-sifted.

The fruits are collected after their full maturation (August – September). They are dried in the shade or the dryer. The dried fruits are red-violet, oval, and wrinkled.

The bark is peeled off in the spring at the start of the juice's movement and is cleared of the cork layer. It is dried in the shade.

The roots are removed in the fall (October) or in the spring (April – May), they are washed, and the thicker pieces are cut and dried in the shade or the dryer.

The entire herb is stored in a dry and well-ventilated area.

What is its chemical composition?

The flowers consist of essential oil, bitter substances, alkaloids, flavonoids, resin, mucilage, tannins, sugar, Vitamin C, organic acids, butter, valeric acid, carotene, iron, malic and tartaric acids, Vitamins from the B group, etc.

 MOTHER'S SECRETS FOR A HEALTHY WINTER

Health Benefits

The flowers act as anti-inflammatory, secretolytic, and expectorant for inflammation of the airways, colds, bronchitis, pneumonia, and cough.

The fruits are slightly laxative, and the leaves – laxative and diuretic.
If you heard before, folk medicine prescribes it for blood pressure, shortness of breath, and difficulty urinating.

The roots and the bark are recommended as a laxative and obesity. Extract from the leaves is used for rheumatism and hemorrhoids. The fruit is used as an immune enhancer and for neuralgia.

You can prepare

You can prepare infusion from the flowers:

2 teaspoons of the herb are covered with 250 ml boiling water. Soak it for 25-30 minutes and from the strained infusion take 2-3 teas a day.

The other way to use it as prevention and treatment for the unwanted flu is to make marvelous Elderberry syrup.

Other uses of the herb

You can make Elderberry Wine (I am sure you heard about it); color your whipped cream or meringues; prepare delicious jelly; fix refreshing chilled juice or the easiest way to try it is to drizzle it on top of your ice-cream 😊.

Health Risk

Please make sure that the berries are ripe and cooked before adding them to your diet.

Also, some people say that we should not give them to small children….

But…. my daughter loves the syrup and I believe
that this little spoon of sweet and aromatic delight
in the morning increases her strength to fight the
colds.

My TradeMark "Immune Bomb":

*And now we reached the time for my
Elderberry Syrup – my "Immune Bomb™":*

*Get 2 cups of dried Elderberries, wash
them well, cover them with 4 cups of cold
water, and add a tablespoon of freshly
grated ginger and one teaspoon of Ceylon
cinnamon powder.*

*Boil the mixture for about an hour or until
the water is half evaporated. Strain it and*

let it cool. To sweeten and supplement with additional healthy benefits of the syrup, add one cup of honey, though you need to ensure that the liquid is lukewarm, not hot.

Keep this fabulous "Immune Bomb™" in glass bottles. Make sure to store it in the refrigerator, so its lifetime increases.

Take one tablespoon per day during the flu period. For the kids, you can give ½ or 1 teaspoon per day, depending on the age. In case this nasty flu enters your home, start taking the regular dosage every 2 hours for the next 2-3 days (not more than 6-8 times daily) and send the cold away.

Flax – Linum Usitatissimun

Imagine pure white and clean bedsheets, feel the crispy, gentle, and smooth touch, and inhale the freshness of the linen……

Elegance and Luxury……

Comfort and Relaxation………

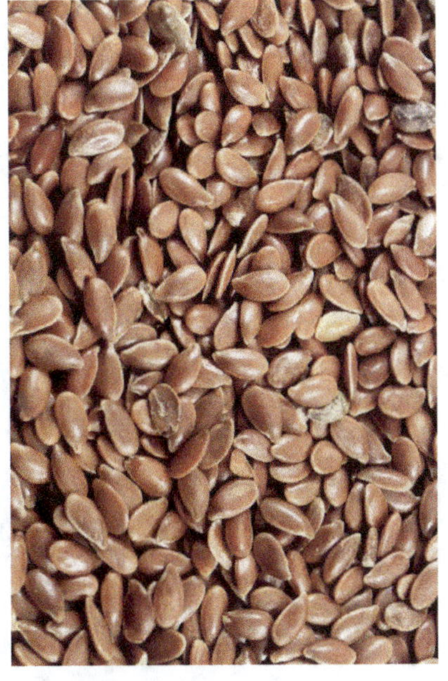

Many thousands of years back, linen fabric was introduced to the world and people made fabulous clothing from the Flax fibers.

But now we are going to concentrate on the Flax seeds because they are one of the pieces in my health puzzle.

Did you know that...

Flax is an annual herbaceous plant with a bare cylindrical stem on top branched, up to 1 ½ meters high.

The leaves resemble lancets and are consistent. The flowers are sky-blue or violet, with handles assembled on top of the stem into thin panicles.

The cup is five-integral, the corolla – five-leaf, and the stamens are five. The fruit is broken into blossom boxes with numerous light brown, shiny seeds.

The Flax plant blooms in June and is wildly cultivated.

As herbs are used the Flax seeds – Semen Lini.

The seeds are harvested at full maturity and dried in the sun or oven. They are rolled, yellow-brown, shiny, odorless, and in mastication have mucus and buttery flavor.

They are preserved in shady, well-ventilated, and dry places.

What is its chemical composition?

The herb has mucilage, contained in the seed shell, so the seeds are extracted whole. Contains pectin, and fatty oils, consisting of glycerides of linoleic, linolenic, isolinolenic, linamarin, proteins, sugars, carotene, etc.

Flaxseeds contain Omega-3, fiber, iron, potassium, Vitamin B1 and B6, magnesium, phosphorus and zinc.

Only good stuff, right?

Health Benefits

If you feel that you need some help with the constipation, then…...

It is better to know that the seeds have a laxative (cleansing) action and mucilaginous (deliquescent the extracts). They increase the volume of fecal matter and thus act purgative.
The seeds are beneficial as well with their anti-inflammatory action. You can use them for inflammatory diseases of the airways (dry cough, bronchial catarrh), of the digestive tract (stomach, intestine), and urinary tract (inflammations and stones in the bladder and kidneys).

Externally you may apply on burns, inflamed mucosa and skin, and swellings….

You can prepare

Crushed Flaxseeds or Flaxseed flour is administered topically in the form of a paw. Mix the herb with hot water, spread it on the gauze, and apply on top of the infected area.

Have Flaxseed oil in your "Medical Cabinet". Works wonders when you mix equal parts of the oil and egg white or lime water and cover burns.

For internal use, Flaxseed is prepared as a cold extract:
1-2 tablespoons seeds and 200 ml cold water. Soak it for 2-3 hours.

OR

Make a potion:

2 tablespoons Flaxseeds and 600 ml boiling water. Boil the mix for 10 minutes. Divide the potion into 6 parts and take 80 ml 15 minutes before and 30 ml after meals.

Other uses of the herb

Flaxseeds are used in the culinary because they are gluten-free and can be combined with other similar flours.

I used them in my granola - mixed with plenty of nuts, other seeds, dried fruits, dates, and oats. My daughter loves it! She takes the granola in a small bowl and eats it dry like she eats nuts.

Sometimes, when I am hungry and there is still time for lunch or dinner, I add one or two tablespoons to a cup of yogurt. It is fulfilling and I love the taste.

Health Risk

Flaxseeds are non-toxic therefore are safe to be used.

Anyway, you better not increase the regular intake, if you wish to reduce your LDL-

Cholesterol levels. Won't go away overnight if you eat 1 kg for dinner……

Everyone's Favorite Yummy Crunchy Granola:

Do you want to make my Yummy Crunchy Granola?

Take 250 g of regular rolled oats,
250 g whole meal oats,
handful of cut into two from each kind of raw nuts: almonds, cashew nuts, hazelnuts
handful of each kind of raw seeds: sunflower, pumpkin, flax, unpeeled sesame
dry fruits as much as you like —banana, papaya, pineapple, coconut (whatever you have at home and you like)
dates – cut into three
Honey – 4-5 tablespoons

Ceylon Cinnamon – 1-2 teaspoons
Ground fresh Ginger

Mix all together without the dates, add some water – just to dampen the oats, drizzle some sunflower oil, and spread on a thin layer in the baking tray. Roast it for 25 - 30 minutes at 150 - 160° C. Stir it regularly to ensure that the mixture is drying up and cooking.

Once you like the color (I prefer to have it brownish for crunchiness) take out the tray and add the dates. Mix well and let it cool.

I am sure that you won't wait till is cool to try. The aroma and the look of it provoke your appetite and you can't stop the mouthwatering……. I know…., it is the same every time at home too.

You can store it in an air-tight jar or container, but the mixture must be cold.

And there you have it - deliciously healthy breakfast, snack, or even before bedtime nibble!

Garlic – Allium Sativum

For sure when you are going to work or getting ready for a "date" after a meal, you prefer to avoid taking a dish that includes this "medicine". Right?

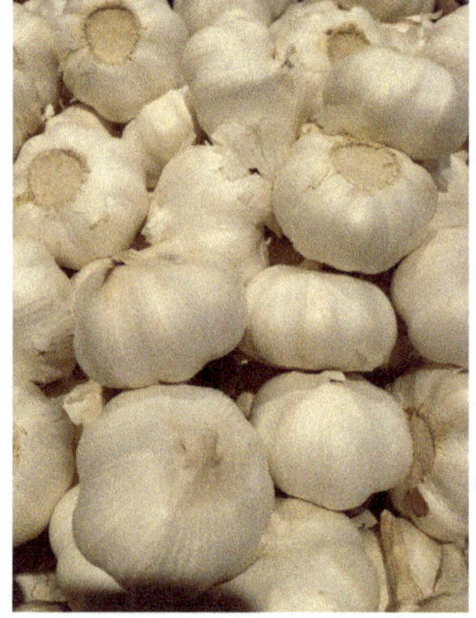

I love to add freshly crushed or grated Garlic in my tomato souse, yogurt salad dressing, mayo or yogurt dips, or even eat the fresh cloves when I eat cooked cabbage for example.

Even the first thing I add to my Quick Fix Cold & Flue Remedy is this fabulous white little "pill".

One of the cheapest and fastest ways to frighten the viruses is to take Garlic. The boyfriend or girlfriend will shrivel his nose if your breath smells of Garlic, but the good news is they are not vampires if they don't run away 😊*.*

Did you know that...

Garlic is a perennial bulbous herb, reaching up to 100 cm in height. It has a complete bulb, which consists of many individual cloves – bulbs.

The inside cloves are oblong and the outside – bold. The whole bulb has a rounded, slightly flattered form in the middle.

The flower stalks near the middle are wrapped with leaves, coming out of the core, and end with a round inflorescence. The leaves are flat, linear, half bent.

The fatherland of the Garlic is South Asia, however is cultivated worldwide.

It is used the bulb of Garlic – Bulbus Allii Sativi.

What is its chemical composition?

The Garlic bulb contains essential oil allicin, which comprises different semi-sulfides. Its main ingredient is dialilsulfid.

During extraction of the herb with water it is produced alliin, which is water soluble and does not possess the odor of Garlic. Under the action of the enzyme aliinaza in the presence of Oxygen from the air (at crushing the bulb), aliinat decays to allicin, and results in its bactericidal action.

The herb consists as well of Vitamin A and B, ferments, iodine, etc.

Health Benefits

The Garlic bulb has versatile accomplishments. Its anthelmintic and its bactericidal action are used for infectious diseases of the gastrointestinal canal.

The essential oil destroys pathogenic and supports the development of normal intestinal flora. It is used in influenza, typhus, and dysentery as a prophylactic.

Stimulates the secretion of gastric and bile juices, and the glands of the digestive tract, and thus improves digestion and the function of the gallbladder.

Part of allicin is emitted through the lungs and acts secretolytic and expectorant is airway inflammation.

You may use it as an excellent prophylactic tool for atherosclerosis.

You can prepare

You can prepare Garlic in the form of gruel (nasal swab) for prophylaxis of flue. Two or three cloves per day are enough for gastrointestinal diseases, loss of appetite, bronchitis, and atherosclerosis……

I use small Garlic cloves to unblock my nose. Sometimes I cover them in tiny pieces of bandage and push them into my nostrils or in my ears. Depending on the intensity of the blockage. If my daughter has a blocked nose and has difficulties breathing, I cut the cloves into smaller pieces, wrap them in the gauze, and leave them in her ears for about 3-5 minutes.

If you wish to remove the unpleasant odor from the Garlic before consumption, take one peeled apple or one tablespoon of honey.

Another way to get rid of the nasty smell is to eat fresh parsley or dill OR drink fresh milk or eat yogurt after enjoying Garlic souse.

Garlic is applied as spirit tincture as well:
Place 50 g crushed Garlic in a dark vessel and cover it with 150 ml 95% alcohol. Soak for 10 days. Take from the tincture 10-15 drops, 3 times per day before meals. If necessary, the drops can be increased or decreased depending on your need.

Other uses of the herb

Cooking of course……. Everyone knows it!

The delightful taste of Garlic and its aroma combined with other lovely herbs and spices can increase your appetite and force you to take one more portion of the marvelous dish, that you or your loved one prepared.

Cosmetics…… You know already that Garlic has an anti-bacterial effect, so you can use it to remove pimples on your skin. Only rub crushed clove onto the affected area and let the magic begin.

I remember when I was younger, with my friends we used to mix up hair masks including Garlic. Brightens and strengthens the hair, and increases the growth because of the calcium and zinc in it and we loved the look of our shiny and long hairs…...

But we waited at least two months before doing any other hair treatments (like waving, straightening, and fixing) in the hair salon. It is very embarrassing if your hairstylist begins to perm your hair and the smell of Garlic fills up the hair salon☹……….

Health Risk

In case you have bleeding disorders or you take blood-thinning medications, please talk to your doctor if you wish to start any treatment with the help of Garlic.

Some people do not tolerate the burning sensation in their mouth or stomach if they eat fresh Garlic.

In this case is better to cook it for a while before consuming it.

There are plenty of ways to include Garlic in your daily diet and today I am not going to give you recipes, because I won't be able to stop writing.

BUT…….

For your next meal, you can prepare Garlic bread. Nothing fancy or difficult. Only cut the bread into slices, and grill them in the oven or the toaster.

While grilling the bread, cut 2-3 cloves of Garlic into two and get the olive oil ready.

Rub Garlic onto the hot bread slices, drizzle olive oil, and season with Himalayan salt and black pepper.

And there you go – you have the most delicious Garlic bread. And you know what? Goes with everything!

Mint – Mentha Piperita

I prefer herbal tea with a soothing taste and natural healing properties.

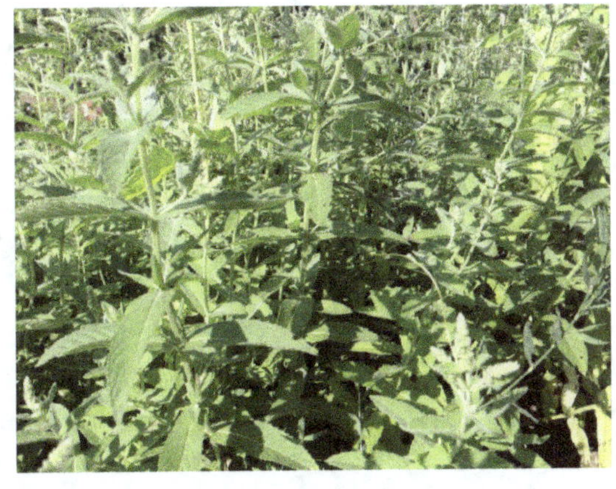

Sometimes I feel like black tea, though……. and the only way to have it is with a pinch of fresh Mint in the pot. These little green leaves carry numerous amounts of freshness and not only the tea pot, but the room is instantly filled with inspirational aroma.

I learned this magical twist from people living in other countries, like the Middle East and North Africa. They prefer black tea, instead of herbal, because they love the strong and saturated taste of caffeine,

     MOTHER'S SECRETS FOR A HEALTHY WINTER

which in some cases can replace morning coffee.

Apologies, I got carried away a little bit.........

Today we are going to talk about the Mint 😊.

Did you know that...

The Mint is a perennial herb with a horizontal rhizome from which grows a few four-keeled and branched stems up to 1 meter high.

The leaves are dark green, with short handles, opposite, oblong, sharply serrated pointed tips, covered with small hairs.

The Mint is small, reddish-purple little flowers, gathered in dense class-prominent inflorescence at the tips of stems.

The fruit consists of four ovate, monocotyledon, reddish-brown wren.

The Mint is a nectariferous plant. The whole plant has a pleasant smell and tastes acrid. The Mint essential oil contains the most valuable ingredient – menthol.

As herbs are used the leaves – Folia Menthae.

The leaves are harvested at the beginning of the flowering (July – August). The entire aboveground part is mowed early in the morning or the evening and the leaves are broken off immediately.

They are spread out in thin layers and dried in the shade or dryer. The dried leaves are dark green on top and light green beneath. They have a peppery taste and aromatic odor.

The leaves are stored in shaded, well-ventilated, and dry places.

What is its chemical composition?

The Mint leaves contain essential oil, which consists of menthol, esters of menthol, cineol, menthen, piperitone; limonene, pulegone, and other terpenes; acetic, isovaleric, and other free acids; methofuran.

The herb consists as well tanning substances, bitter substances, nicotinic acid, caffeic and chlorogenic acid, and flavone glycosides.

Health Benefits

Peppermint oil in small doses increases appetite, works well when feeling sick, and relieves spasms, especially colic in the stomach, intestines, and bile duct, the gases expelled in flatulence. Excites the extraction of the liver and pancreas and acts astringent and anti-inflammatory.

Because of these actions, the herb is good in the treatment of functional disorders of the stomach, chronic pancreatitis, indigestion, nausea, vomiting, and diarrhea.

The menthol induces reflex expansion of the coronary vessels. You may use it as well as antiseptic, analgesic, and in inflammatory diseases of the upper respiratory tract – take it internally or in the form of inhalation.

You can prepare peppermint oil in an alcohol solution and use it as a local antiseptic to treat neurodermatitis.

The folk medicine recommends the Mint leaves to cure dizziness, insomnia, headache, melancholy, epilepsy…... Decoction of the leaves are great treat in the form of a bath for nervous conditions or used to gargle for sore gums, toothaches, and bad breath.

You can prepare

Take the herb internally as an infusion:

Cover 2 teaspoons of Mint leaves with 200 ml boiling water. Allow to soak for 20 minutes, then strain and the infusion take in small sips 3 times a day, 200 ml each time, 1 hour after meal.

Other uses of the herb

Cosmetics – toothpaste, creams, shampoos, conditioners, perfumes, air fresheners….

Culinary – salads, cooked dishes, sauces, creams, cakes, liquors, soft drinks, candies, chewing gums, garnish…...

It is used also as "organic insecticide" – sends away (and kills) the unwanted wasps and ants.

Health Risk

Although Mint is safe, might cause allergic reactions. Please do not overdose on the internal intake and NEVER take internally the essential oil. Pure menthol is toxic and poisonous.

DO NOT apply Mint oil on the face of a small child, because may cause difficulty in breathing and spasms.

Today I will give you two ideas including Mint – one for lunch and the other one for an afternoon drink…….

My Delicious Spring Green Rice Recipe:

You need 1 teacup of rice (it is better to be short grain), 12-15 spring onions, 2-3 tablespoons of olive oil, ½ bunch of dill, ½ bunch of mint leaves, 3-4 tea cups of vegetable bouillon (depends on the rice), Himalayan salt, black pepper.

Chop the spring onions and braise in the oil. Once they are soft, add the rice. Simmer for 1-2 minutes, until the rice becomes transparent. Poor 1 cup of the broth and simmer, while stirring occasionally. When the rice almost absorbed the broth, add one more cup. Then one more cup and the salt and pepper too.

When the rice is almost done, and there is still a little bit of broth unabsorbed, add the chopped dill and mint leaves. Stir again and remove from the stove. Cover with a lid and let it rest for 20 minutes.

The result is amazingly tasty rice. The onions won't taste very strongly and the fresh herbs complement the smoothness of the rice. You can enjoy it as a main dish, on the other hand, you may serve it as a side dish along with roasted meat or chicken.

AND

The Delightful & Refreshing Minty Lemonade:

Take ½ a coffee cup of sugar, add it to a saucepan with 1 coffee cup of water, bring to a boil, and let it boil for 2-3 minutes. Stir it occasionally to ensure that the sugar dissolves well. Let it cool.

Squeeze 6-7 lemons and pour the juice into the blender, add a handful of fresh mint leaves, 2 tea cups of water, half of the sugar syrup, and ice if you like. Mix well.

Serve in a chilled glass, decorated with lemon slices and fresh mint leaves. Have on the side the other half of the sugar syrup, some lemon juice, slices of lemon, and mint leaves. If you wish to balance the

   MOTHER'S SECRETS FOR A HEALTHY WINTER

sweetness, sourness, and freshness to your taste you can add in the glass.

Enjoy this full of coolness and energy lemonade!

Oregano – Origanum Vulgare

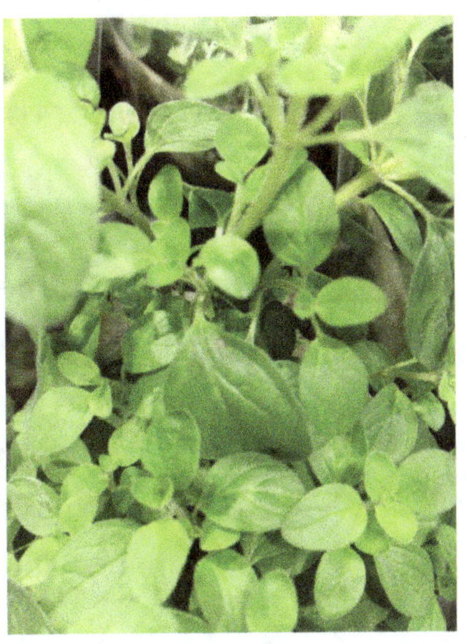

Did you know that the name in Greek means mountain happiness and Oregano is mentioned in the books of Virgil and Aristotle? The ancient Greek philosopher wrote how wounded with an arrow chamois hurry to eat the fragrant grass and to save their lives.

Even wild animals know that this miraculous plant is a fertile offspring of nature.

I love to prepare Oregano tea upon the first signs of cold or flu or even if I feel like having something hot and aromatic to drink.

Did you know that...

The Oregano is a perennial herbaceous plant with a straight four-ribbed stem up to 1 meter high, branched at the top, rarely haired.

The leaves are relatively small, with a whole leaf edge, opposite, ovate, with short handles, slightly or heavily hairy, and the lower leaves are larger.

The flowers are located on top of the stem, gathered in spikes arranged as panicles in the bosom of tile-shaped bracts.
The bract leaves are purple, and the flowers – pink. The cup and the bracts have oil glands. The fruit crumbles in four wrens.

You can find Oregano among bushes, on stony meadows, in clearings and forests.

For herb is used the shoot of the Oregano – Herba Origani.

The overhead of the plant is collected during the flowering (June – July). The stems are cut 20 cm from the top, and then they are knotted into small bushes and dried in the shade or dryer.

Well-dried herb has a slightly bitter taste. It is stored in shaded and well-ventilated areas.

What is its chemical composition?

The Oregano contains essential oils – thymol, carvacrol, geranilacitat, tannins, bitter substance, carotene, vitamin C, etc....

Health Benefits

I am sure you heard before that Oregano has diverse actions. Supports expectoration and calms the cough, acts as well for acute and chronic bronchitis.

Will help you remove the spasms in the stomach, painful menstruation, and liver inflammation.

Improves digestion and increases appetite, stimulates peristalsis, and has a favorable effect on dyspnea and jaundice. It is common in increasing diuresis.

You can prepare

If you wish to use the herb externally, you may do it in the form of baths for rashes, lichens, or itchy eczema. For baths, you should prepare an infusion of 200-300 grams of herb and 2-3 liters of boiling water.

For internal use, make the following infusion: Brew 1-2 tablespoons finely chopped Oregano with 400 ml boiling water. Soak it for 30 minutes and take from it 3 times a day.

For sure you can make tea if you like.

Other uses of the herb

Culinary of course! This is the best way to add it to your diet. Enhance the taste of your salad, soup, or meat dish with a pinch of fresh or dried Oregano.
The essential oil is a good remedy against moths and ants 😉.

Health Risk

Be careful while giving it to your kids too – disregard the essential oil, especially for kids under 2, and avoid or reduce the portions of Oregano tea or infusions to 1/3 of the normal dose for colds and coughs. For bigger children, you can use ½ to full of the regular dosage, depending on the age.
Like with all herbs, please be alert if you have any allergies or you are pregnant, because of the possibility of bleeding.

The Heavenly Roasted Veggies:

Do you feel like having Roasted Veggies with Oregano today?

See how you can make them:

Prepare 2 big ripped tomatoes, 2 big pilled potatoes, 2-3 handfuls of mushrooms, 3-4 teaspoons of olive oil, Himalayan salt, black pepper, and the herb of the Day – 1 teaspoon of fresh Oregano leaves (or dry if that's what you have at home).

Cut the tomatoes into 1 cm round slices, and the potatoes and the mushrooms into thin round slices. Cover the cooking tray with 1-2 spoons of olive oil, place the potatoes and the mushrooms on the bottom, and then cover with the tomato slices.

Season with salt, pepper, and Oregano and drizzle the remaining oil on top.

Cook in the oven for about 30 – 40 minutes at 180 C. If you wish to add grated cheese on top, do it 10 minutes before removing the dish from the oven, so the cheese melts and gets brownish and crispy.

You can serve this Veggie-Oregano Delight as a main or side dish.

OR

The Irresistible Recharging & Aromatic Bath:

Maybe you are feeling tired and prefer to recharge your energy in an aromatic bath……Oregano is the right tool to help you achieve the best refreshing and stimulating effect.

Take 100 grams of Oregano and cover it with 1 liter boiling water. Simmer for 10 minutes, and then leave it to soak for 10 more minutes. Strain and add to your bathtub filled with 2/3 warm water.

It is enough to dive in this marvelously fragrant water and within 15 minutes to feel the energy and good mood entering your entire body and mind.

Your choice……., however, enjoy it!

Rosemary – Rosmarinus Officinalis

Its unforgettable fragrance mixed between pine and spices, brings a sense of forest and sea....

The other names of the Rosemary are "The Sea Dew" and "Sea Rose" and many parents decided to name their baby girl after this amazing herb 😊.

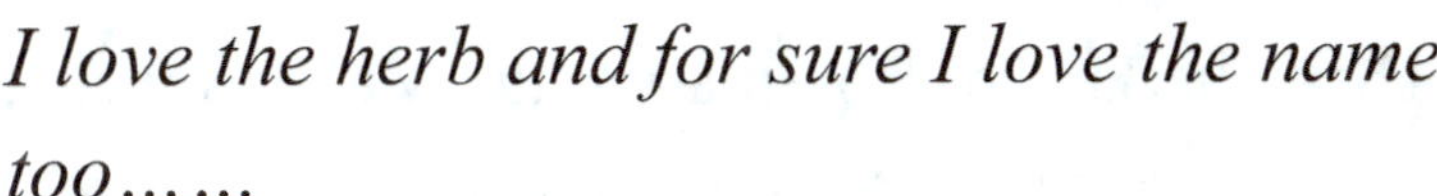

I love the herb and for sure I love the name too……

Did you know that...

Rosemary is a perennial plant of the family Lamiaceae and is available throughout the year.

Its leaves resemble needles of pine trees – long and narrow with a pointed tip. They are dark green on the outside and silver-white on the inside. The length of the leaves is between 2 and 4 cm and their width is between 2 and 5 cm.

I enjoy looking at the blooming beautiful flowers of the plant. The colors are different and in the gentle baby nuances – pink, purple, white, and blue.

I have a Rosemary shrub near the barbeque/summer kitchen area and only glancing from time to time at it helps me prepare lovely meals.

The fatherland of Rosemary is the Mediterranean, which gives its sensation of the sea.

Rosemary flowers during spring and summer in mild regions however may blooms throughout the year in places with warm climates.

As herbs are used the Rosemary leaves.

If possible, use the fresh Rosemary leaves, because they have with better taste and more intense flavor, than the dried leaves. Fresh Rosemary leaves should be dark green and without yellow or dark spots.

Fresh Rosemary leaves you can store in the refrigerator in slightly damp paper/kitchen towel or the best is to have the Rosemary grown in a pot and use it throughout the year.

Dried Rosemary is widely used too, however, make sure you store it in an airtight container in a dark, cool, and dry place.

What is its chemical composition?

Rosemary is a great source of vitamin A, vitamin C, calcium, iron, magnesium, carotenoids, rosmarinic acid, carnosol, camphor, etc.

Health Benefits

If you have any respiratory issues or often you encounter asthma attacks, count on its anti-inflammatory compounds and you will find that Rosemary reduces the attacks. Will help you remove infections of the ear, nose, and throat.

Rosemary contains substances that help the immune system and improve blood circulation as well. The herb is an excellent antioxidant that is packed with flavonoids regulates the thyroid gland and relieves headache.

One more curiously interesting action of the Rosemary is that improves concentration, and memory and increases the blood flow to the brain. This is the reason that the ancient Greek students used to decorate their hair with Rosemary twigs when they studied for examinations.

Rosemary helps digestion too. If you suffer from stomach problems or bloating, Rosemary easily can handle them. Also helps rapid weight loss.

Honesty, I did not use the herb for that reason, but the fact that improves the digestion is good enough for me to accept that Rosemary helps us release the toxins.

You can prepare

If you have dandruff, prepare an infusion from Rosemary and rinse the hair every time after washing it with shampoo.

To prepare the infusion: take 2 tablespoons of Rosemary leaves (fresh or dried) and cover with 400 ml boiling water. Simmer for 5 minutes in low heat, leave for 15 minutes to soak, and then strain the infusion.
Rosemary oil is good for skin rashes and eczema. Simply rub the affected area with a small cotton pad dipped in organic Rosemary oil and see the rush go away in 1-2 days.

You can prepare Rosemary tincture too:
Mix ½ cup of vodka or rubbing alcohol with 1 tablespoon of Rosemary leaves. Leave the

mixture for 10 days and then strain. You can dilute 20 drops of the tincture in 20-30 ml water every morning and drink it before breakfast.

The fragrant tasty Rosemary tea is an excellent remedy if you catch a cold or you feel depressed……

Other uses of the herb

Of course, in Culinary is the main use of Rosemary – fresh and dry leaves. Goes excellent with any meat – roasted or stewed, salad dressings, and fresh or grilled vegetables.

Cosmetics! Rosemary oil is used in shampoos, hair conditioners, perfumes, and air fresheners.

Religious applications…. Rosemary twigs can be thrown into the grave of the deceased as a symbol of remembrance.

I love my Rosemary pots around the house. And they return their love to me with aromatic help,

while protecting the area from the insects J.
Simply said – I use the Rosemary as a pest
deterrent.

Health Risk

The herb is mild and does not have any allergens,
however, be cautious with the use of Rosemary
during pregnancy.

It is difficult to overdose with the herb, because
of the strong flavor, but you still need to be
careful not to spoil your meal.

My Easy To Enhance Olive Oil Recipe:

*Today I will not tell you to do something
difficult……*

*The easiest way to enhance your olive oil is
to add one sprig of fresh Rosemary into the
bottle and voila – you've got the most
aromatic oil for your salads.*

Scotch Pine – Pinus Silvestris

I like the smell of fresh green pine brunches. Reminds me of Christmas and the busy preparations for the Holiday season.

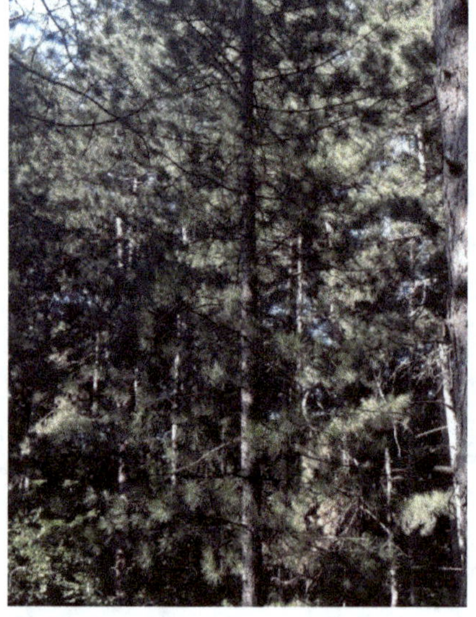

Maybe you heard before that the Native Americans opened up the secret to the European people, living in North America, that to fight the colds and winter diseases, they should chew and even eat the Pine needles………....

Did you know that...

White Pine is an evergreen, resinous, monoecious tree, reaching a height of 30 m. The bark on the lower part is grey and cracked, and the top – light brown.

The leaves are needle-like placed by two and are rounded outside, but inward recessed with membranous scales at the base.

Male flowers are yellow catkins and are collected in many false bunches of stamens and two anthers.

Female flowers are collected in ovate cones at the tips of young twigs and consist of red flakes, the base of which has two ovules.

The cones grow after coaters. They ripen after the second year and their scales open and the seeds fall off.

The Pine blooms in May – June.

As herbs are used the Pine buds – Tiriones Pini. Besides the buds are used also the Pine bark and the wood chips, Pine balm, the essential oil from the Pine needles and the twigs Pine juice, and the oil from the seeds.

The Pine buds are harvested in early spring when they begin to open up. They are the main herb used for herbal treatments.

They are almost cylindrical, long 2-5 cm, and thick 4 mm. They consist of the axis, around which are densely arranged numerous black-brown scales, colorless and torn around the edge, and glued with a resinous secretion. In the bosom of each flake is one ovule.

The Pine buds are dried in the shade or a dryer. Afterwards, the herb is packed in bags. The dried herb is with pinkish-brown color with a pleasant balsamic smell and resin-bitter taste.

What is its chemical composition?

The buds contain essential oil, vitamins B1, C, and K, tannins, resinous substances, carotene, and others.

The essential oil contains mainly α-pinene, less β-pinene, dipentene, terpineol, ladinen, limonene, borneol, complex esters, and free alcohols.

Health Benefits

The Pine tops are excellent as antiseptic in acute and chronic bronchitis, tonsillitis, and inflammation of the upper respiratory tract, because they act as softener of the mucous membrane.

I usually use them in the form of inhalation and rubbing.

The essential oil derived from the resin of the white pine is used in diseases of the bronchi and the lungs. It has bacterial properties; it acts as a diuretic; urinary dissolves kidney stones and cleanses the bladder.

The essential oil is used for threatening eczemas, lichens, and rashes due to its action to dilate blood vessels and warm the skin.

Due to its anti-inflammatory action has a good effect on rheumatism, stabbing, lumbago, neuralgia, and gout.

The folk medicine recommends it for shortness of breath, edema, and scurvy.

From the Pine buds, I often prepare honey syrup to treat colds and bronchitis. Sometimes I prepare baths with the buds to prevent rheumatism and relieve skin rashes.

You can prepare

You can prepare decoction from Pine buds:
Cover 1 tablespoon Pine tops with 300 ml boiling water and simmer for about 1 minute. Leave it to soak for 30 minutes, strain, and sweeten if you wish with honey. You, as an adult can drink 80 ml from the decoction, 3 times a day before meals; to

your kids, though you may give only up to 40 ml at the time, 3 times per day before meals.

The syrup is easy to make too……….. Cover 50 g of chopped Pine tops with 500 ml boiling water. Mix well and let it cool. Once cools down to room temperature, strain and add 700 – 800 g honey, then mix until the honey dissolves well. Take 1 tablespoon (1 teaspoon for the kid) 3-4 times a day before meals.

Remember I mentioned previously that if you suffer from bronchitis or any lung disease, you can do inhalations?
Boil 2 l of water and add 5 drops of essential oil from Pine buds. Inhale for 10 minutes and feel the relief 😊.

If you have rheumatism or you have any skin disease, the best way to treat them is to prepare baths. Take 500 g Pine tops, boil them in 5 l water for 30 minutes, and add the strained extract to your bathtub.

 MOTHER'S SECRETS FOR A HEALTHY WINTER

Other uses of the herb

The essential oil is widely used in the cosmetic industry – face creams, soaps, shampoos, conditioners, air fresheners, detergents……...
My mother for example uses the broken Pine brunches from the trees in her courtyard and places them in the fireplace during the autumn. They burn fast and develop high temperatures and of course, the room gets warm quicker. And the aroma is amazing – no need for an air freshener……...

Health Risk

As with any other herb, the higher doses may irritate the mucous membrane of the stomach and the intestines, and cause depression or insomnia.

Please do not use the herb if you are pregnant or you have an inflammatory process in your kidney parenchyma.

Contact your doctor before deciding to begin home treatment with the herb.

The Exceptional 5 Steps Exercise To Heal Your Lungs:

Today you will learn the recipe for the easiest exercise ever………… Only 5 steps:

1. *Get out and find a Pine nearby.*
2. *Inhale that magical Pine fragrance.*
3. *Fill up your lungs with a healing, spiritual, and nourishing aroma.*
4. *Let your mind relax and enjoy the feeling.*
5. *Thank nature for this amazing gift and be blessed.*

Thyme – Thymus Sp. Diversae (T. Serpyllum)

Thyme is one of my favorite herbs and spices of course.

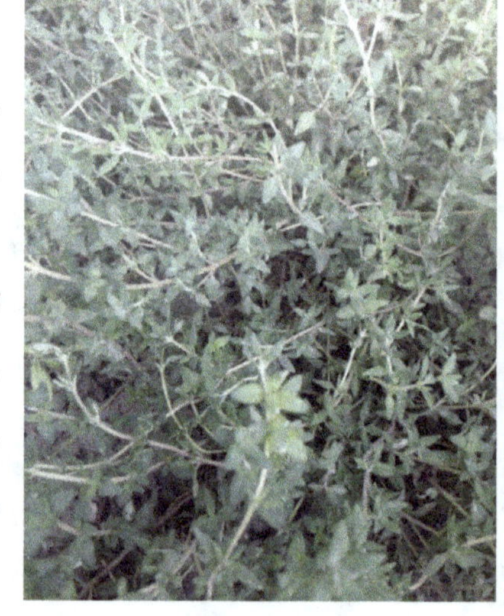

These little pinkish or violet flowers and the tiny delicate leaves are soooooo aromatic and memorable that I use them for almost every meat dish and even for salads.

The great thing is that is available all year round and I truly enjoy adding it to my meals and teas.

Thyme is a fragrant herb with many health benefits and today I am happy to share my "Thyme Experience" with you.

Did you know that...

The Thyme is a perennial plant with creeping stems, which grow several raised or crawling, bare, or hairy branches.

The leaves are opposite, oval egg-shaped to narrowly lanceolate, rounded at the tip, and narrowed at the base to about 3 cm long handle.

The lamina is about 0.5 – 1.5 cm long and 7 mm wide, without a pointed down edge with cilia at the base.

The upper surface of the leaves has a greenish-grey color and the bottom is whitish.

The flowers are collected together at the tips of stems in prolonged or intermittent inflorescences.

The cup is green, sometimes reddish, bilabial. The corolla is pale pink or red, with unclear bilabial, with incised upper and tripartite lower lip. Stamens are four.

The fruit is composed of four spherical nuts.

All above-ground parts of the Thyme are covered with essential oil glands, which seem dashed-line against the light.

The plant has a pleasant characteristic odor. Blooms all summer.

You easily can find Thyme near forests, meadows, roads and rocks, and sunny places.

For herbs is used the overhead part – Herba Thymi.

The ground part of the plant is harvested during flowering (May – September), by cutting with a knife or scissors. It is dried in the shade or dryer. The dried herb has a light brown stem.

The cup and the leaves are green, and the fruits are pink-red or violet with a pleasant aroma and slightly bitter taste.

You may store it in a shady, well-ventilated, and dry place.

What is its chemical composition?

The Thyme contains about 1% essential oil – composition of p-cymene, carvacrol, thymol, borneol, geraniol, linalool, tannins, flavone glycosides, mineral salts, bitter substance – serpilin, and others.

Health Benefits

Thyme is famous for its pectolytic, expectorant in catarrh of the upper respiratory tract, chronic bronchitis, flu, and inflammation of the lungs with mucus secretions.

I am confident that at least once before you used Thyme to soothe your dry and spasmodic cough, right?!

Thyme oil has antioxidant and antimicrobial properties and over and over again is used to fight against different bacteria and fungi.

Often is prescribed as a nerve sedative and antispasmodic for stomach and intestinal diseases, mainly with nervous origin – chronic gastritis, ulcers, headaches, radiculitis, and neuritis.

Sometimes I use it to prepare aromatic baths and compresses if I feel any irritation and I need an analgesic agent for my muscles and my joints.

The most I use it for my cough syrups and teas during the winter and when the nasty flu is everywhere around us.

And of course, I use it for my Rubbing Thyme Ointment. The best way to relieve the blocked nose and remove the cold from my daughter's chest.

You can prepare

The folk medicine recommends Thyme as well for anorexia, insomnia, rheumatism, and gargling for inflammations of the lining of the mouth and throat.

You can prepare decoction and infusion from the Thyme.

Decoction: Take 2 tablespoons of the herb and cover it with 400 ml boiling water. Boil it for 3 minutes, and then soak for 1 hour and strain. From the decoction take 120 ml, 3 times a day.

Infusion: Cover 2 tablespoons of the herb with 500 ml boiling water and let it soak for 2 hours. From the infusion take 4 times a day, 100 ml each time.

If you need to use the herb externally, then prepare an infusion from 100 g of the herb and 2 liters of boiling water. Allow it to stay for 30 minutes, strain it, and add to the water in your bathtub.

Other uses of the herb

For thousands of years various herbs and spices have been used in food storage or to protect the foods from microbial contamination. Thyme is one of these special herbs 😊.

You can add Thyme – fresh or dry to your salads, to your roasted meat or chicken, to your cheese or vegetables, egg omelet, or steamed rice 😉.

And of course, the Thyme oil is great if you add it to your massage oil. You are going to benefit from it completely – aroma therapy that will open up your skin pores, relieve the stiff muscles, remove any skin irritation, unclog your lungs and nose, and relax your soul and mind.

If you never tried it before, simply do it! And trust me – you are going to love it.

Health Risk

Thyme is safe when consumed in normal amounts of food and in this form can be taken by children and pregnant and nursing mothers.

Thyme oil in small quantities is safe as well, however, please be careful if you take any blood clotting medications, like aspirin, ibuprofen, etc., because Thyme has a similar effect and a higher dosage may increase the chances of bleeding.

As usual, please consult your doctor, if you wish to incorporate Thyme in your home remedies.

The Proven "Rubbing Cold Removing Ointment":

Today we are going to prepare my Rubbing Thyme Ointment

You may know already that ointments are made to form a film on top of the skin and protect it from further damage.

Anyway, I am fixing my ointment a little bit more liquefied, so can be absorbed through the skin and reach and release the nasty mucus from the lungs and nose.

Usually, the ointments are made from 1 cup of infused oil and 1 block (1 oz) of beeswax. I will add 2-3 tablespoons of coconut butter and 1 teaspoon of lavender oil.

OK, let's start:

Mix the infused oil, the beeswax, and the coconut butter in a glass bowl, which is part of your double boiler. If you don't have a double boiler, then use any glass or ceramic bowl that fits in a saucepan filled with water. The idea is to use the steam and heat the mixture in your bowl, without overheating the ingredients.

Melt the mix at a low temperature and stir it with a wooden or ceramic spoon. Once all ingredients are melted gradually, remove from the heat and add your favorite essential oil.
Then pour the obtained liquid into a glass jar with a lid. I usually use a few small jars, because it is easier to use them later on and at the same time the small doses increase the ointment life.

Close the jar and keep it in the fridge. May last for 3 – 4 months.

I am sure that you will love the smell and most importantly – the healing results 😊*.*

Tilia – Tili Argentea, Tilia Cordata, Tilia Platyphyllos

Tilia or Linden or Lime Tree or Basswood………

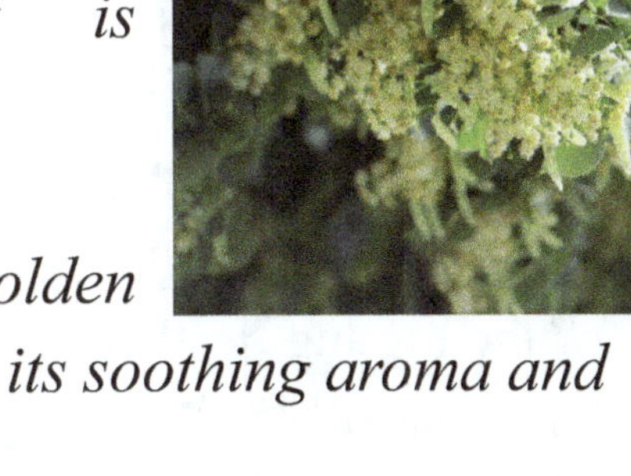

Whichever name you know or you choose, the healing effect of this miraculous plant is proven.

I love the pinkish-golden color of the tea and its soothing aroma and charming taste.

Did you know that...

Today we are going to talk about the three types of Tilia – Silver Linden, Small-Leaved, and Large-Leaved Linden.

They are trees, 20 – 30 meters high, with wildly branched dense crowns.

The leaves are consistent with long petioles, irregularly heart-shaped tapered, and unevenly serrated at their base stipules.

The leaves of the small-leaf Linden are dark green on top, the bottom is bluish-green, and the angles between the streaks on the lower side are strigose with yellow-red hairs.

The flowers are collected in a semi-hood whose handle to about half its connate with the main vein of the big lug, leathery, with a net of lines bract that in small-leaf and large-leaf is naked and in silver-leaf is whitish hairy.

The flowers are yellowish-white.

The cup in all species is five-leaf, and the corolla is not accreted. The stamens are many. The small-leaf Linden blossom in the middle of summer, before large-leaf and silver-leaf Linden.

The leaves of the large-leaf Linden are equal green from both sides; the angles between the lines on the lower side are strigose with whitish hairs. The flowers are light yellow.

For herbs, the flower of the Linden–Flores Tiliae.

The flowers of the Linden tree are harvested with or without bract. They are harvested during the flowering (July – August). First blooms the small-leaf Linden, and later the silver-leaf Linden.

Picking up the flowers is done carefully – if they crush and straticulate may cause them to brew and while drying, they darken. They are dried in the shade or a dryer.

You will know that the herb is dry when the flower handles while bending them begin to break.

After drying the herb should be protected from the effects of direct sunlight, because they fade. The dry flower is light yellow and has a yellowish-green stipule, pleasant smell, and sweet-bitter taste.

It is stored in shaded and well-ventilated areas.

What is its chemical composition?

The Linden flowers contain essential oil with the main ingredient sesquiterpene alcohol, mucilage, tannins, flavonoids, talipot, chlorogenic, caffeic and coumaric acid, saponins, carotene, vitamin C, etc.

Health Benefits

The main effect of the Linden flower is diaphoretic, antipyretic, and diuretic.

It is excellent for treating flu, bronchial catarrh, angina, and pneumonia, any temperature conditions, inflammation of the kidneys and bladder, urethritis.

Maybe you heard before that it is prescribed as an anti-inflammatory agent in inflammation of the upper respiratory tract and functional disorders of the stomach and intestines.

Linden flower has sedative and antispasmodic action too.

Falk medicine is recommended for dizziness, epilepsy, skin rashes, headaches, and hysteria.

You can prepare

If you have any throat infection or inflammation of the oral cavity, use it as a gargle. If you experience any neurosis, add strong infusion into your bathtub.

For internal use you can make infusion from Linden flower:
2 – 3 teaspoons herb and 250 ml boiling water. Allow to soak for 20 minutes, strain and drink at once.

Other uses of the herb

Because of its incredible fragrance, Linden is used for perfume making and cosmetic creams too.

The bees are very clever beings and recognize the greatness of the Linden as well. They use the Linden nectar to create their outstanding Linden honey.

Linden is used in culinary as well – creams, syrups, and sweet cheese flavored with its amazing blossoms.

Health Risk

Most of the parts of the Linden tree are eatable and with soothing effect.
If you have any doubts, please contact your doctor before adding the Linden to your diet.

My Grandmother's Astonishing Linden
Syrup:

*Take around 25 Linden blossom clusters
with some open and some still closed buds.
From these clusters remove the flowers.
You should get around 8 – 9 handfuls of
Linden blossom. Wash them well.*

*Place the Linden flowers in a clean glass
container and cover on top with lemon zest
and lemon juice from 2 lemons.*

*In different pots prepare sugar syrup – into
one liter of water add 500 – 600g sugar.
Boil the water until the sugar dissolves
well. Let it cool a bit and add 1 – 2 cups of
honey. Stir the mixture well.*

*Pour the sugar syrup over the bed of Linden
Lemon Zest and cover the container. Let it*

rest for one day, then transfer the container to the fridge.

If you believe you won't be able to finish the syrup in one month, add some citric acid (1 tablespoon) when you mix all the ingredients.

After 4 days strain the syrup and store it in glass bottles in the refrigerator.

From My Grandmother's Linden Syrup, I make summer refreshing chilled juice:
In a 1-liter glass jar pour 100ml of the syrup, add ice cubes, fill up with water, and a few slices of lemon. Mix well and serve in chilled glasses.

You may add more syrup if you wish 😊

Conclusion

That was my story and my experience with different herbs, which helped me and my family stay healthy and energized throughout the year.

We use the food and the plants to keep our bodies strong and well. Instead of medical tablets and chemical syrups, I prepare natural candies, syrups, marmalades, and refreshing teas.

I hope that you enjoyed my simple book and that you followed every "exercise" after the introduction of each magical herb. I hope that I helped you to find better ways to keep your family away from diseases…...

I wish you all the health, love, positive energy, and abundance in the world to flow into your home, embrace You and Your family, and stay there FOREVER

"The doctor of the future will no longer treat the human frame with drugs, but rather will Cure and prevent disease with nutrition." Thomas Edison

---

THE END